Healthy eating

No matter who you a
fact that you are aliv
keeping hydrated. A
be one of the most sa

and can also be responsible for some of our greatest
health problems.

You are essentially what you eat. Each human
being is made up of water, protein, fat, minerals and
vitamins. Every single molecule comes from the food
you eat and the water you drink. Eating the highest
quality food in the right quantities helps you to
achieve your highest potential for health, vitality and
freedom from disease.

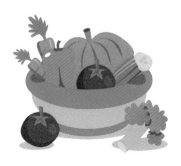

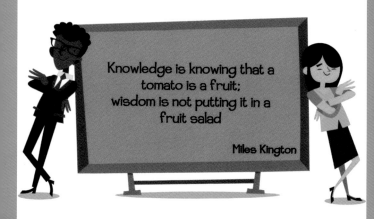

Knowledge is knowing that a tomato is a fruit;
wisdom is not putting it in a fruit salad

Miles Kington

This bite-sized book has been designed to offer a useful overview for everyone about healthy eating and help achieve the following:

- Understand the benefits of healthy eating
- Establish ways to maintain a balanced diet
- Raise awareness of each of the food groups
- Energise yourself through what you consume
- Fuel your immune system for well-being

Please note that the content in this book is not intended to replace the advice of a doctor or any other specialist health professional or practitioner. Any statistics used within have been sourced from the WHO (World Health Organization).

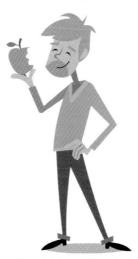

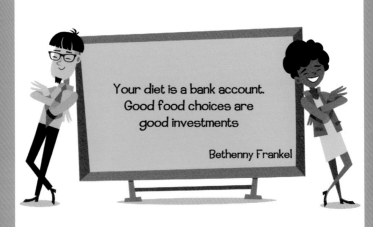

Your diet is a bank account.
Good food choices are
good investments

Bethenny Frankel

Understanding food

How many times have you followed a diet without really understanding the difference between a protein and a complex carbohydrate?

Understanding the food groups and the benefits of what each of them do is a useful place to start. Here is a basic low-down on which nutrients are found in what.

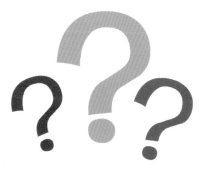

Proteins

Proteins are made up of many building blocks, known as amino acids. All cells and tissues in your body contain protein, therefore protein is essential for growth and repair and the maintenance of good health. Different foods contain different amounts and combinations of amino acids.

You will be able to consume protein from animal sources including meat, fish, eggs and dairy products which contain the full range of essential amino acids needed for the healthy function of your body. Vegans and vegetarians can also get all the amino acids they need by combining different plant sources of protein including pulses and cereals.

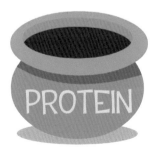

Carbohydrates

Carbohydrates are neutral compounds of carbon, hydrogen and oxygen. Carbohydrates come in simple forms such as sugars and in complex forms such as starches and fibre.

Carbohydrates are all about energy and are found in foods like fruits, vegetables, breads, pasta and dairy products. Your body uses these foods to make glucose, which is your body's main energy source. Carbohydrates provide the body with the energy it needs and are a good source of many vitamins and minerals too.

There are two main types of carbohydrates: complex and simple. Complex carbohydrates are those in whole grain, and simple carbohydrates are those that are refined and have been processed and broken down.

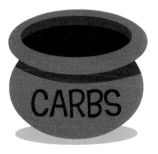

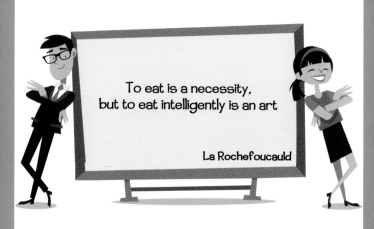

To eat is a necessity,
but to eat intelligently is an art

La Rochefoucauld

Everything in moderation

Understanding yourself and discovering what works best for you is the first step to better health and personal performance. There are, however, some key aspects of nutrition that are fundamental to everyone and it is helpful to understand what healthy eating is all about.

Occasionally, you may want to enjoy treats and there is, of course, a lot of temptation about. It is important however, that the underpinning framework for your lifestyle is a well-balanced one. Successful lifestyle management is all about the healthy choices you make and enjoying everything in moderation.

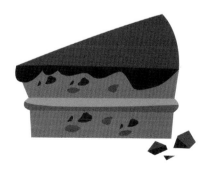

Fats

Fats and oils are both concentrated sources of energy. Some have health benefits in moderation and some do not. Eating too much of the wrong kinds of fat, like saturated and industrially-produced trans-fat, can increase the risk of heart disease and stroke and various other illnesses.

Unsaturated vegetable oils including olive, soy, sunflower or corn oil are the healthier alternative to animal fats or any oils that are high in saturated fats which include butter, ghee, lard, coconut and palm oil. To avoid unhealthy weight gain, consumption of total fat should not exceed 30% of your overall energy intake.

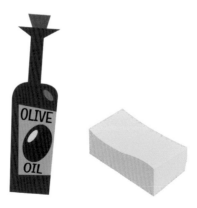

Fibre

The ideal intake is not less than 35 grams a day. It is relatively easy to take in this amount of fibre. The fibre you consume absorbs water into the digestive tract making the food contents bulkier and easier to pass through the body.

A great way to absorb fibre is eating whole grains, vegetables, fruit, nuts and seeds on a daily basis. Cereal fibre and linseed are especially good for avoiding constipation.

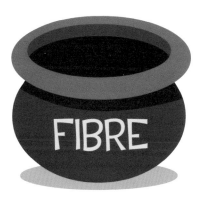

Vitamins

Although required in smaller amounts than fats, proteins or carbohydrates, vitamins are extremely important to our diets. They stimulate enzymes which in turn make all the body processes happen.

Vitamins are needed to balance hormones, produce energy, boost the immune system, make healthy skin and protect our arteries. They are also vital for our brain, nervous system and just about every bodily function.

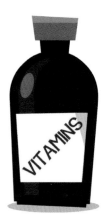

Minerals

Like vitamins, minerals are essential too. Calcium, magnesium and phosphorus help make up the bones and teeth. Nerve signals, which are vital for the brain and muscles, depend on calcium, magnesium, sodium and potassium.

Other minerals include chromium for controlling blood sugar levels and selenium and zinc which are essential for bodily repair and the immune system.

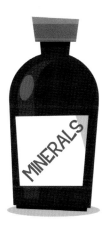

A healthy balanced diet

A well-balanced diet along with physical activity are the foundations of good health. Healthy eating is about consuming high-quality proteins, carbohydrates, heart-healthy fats, vitamins, minerals and water. It is important to minimise processed foods, saturated fats and alcohol. This approach will help you to maintain your body's everyday functions, maintain optimal body weight and also help with disease prevention.

Here are some useful tips and advice that will help you to look after your overall well-being and feel more energised:

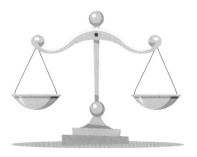

How to fuel yourself well

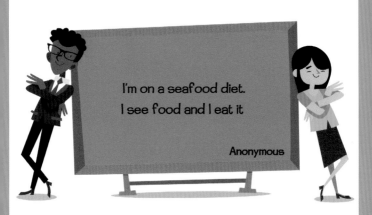

I'm on a seafood diet.
I see food and I eat it

Anonymous

Eating and lifestyle

It is really important to get into some good habits around food so that you can create a healthy lifestyle. Here are some ways to make healthy changes in your eating habits:

- Wherever possible eat your meals at the table rather than in bed, at your desk or sitting on the sofa watching TV.
- Eat mindfully and savour the experience.
- Cook from scratch and have takeaways as an occasional treat only.
- Chew some gum when you cook so you are not tempted to snack on the ingredients.
- Keep a tub of ready chopped fruit and vegetables to snack on when you feel the urge to reach for a quick fix.
- Pack a healthy lunch and snacks for work as this will give you more control over what you eat.
- Put your snacks on a plate instead of eating from the packet and this will help you control how many you eat.
- Avoid skipping or delaying meals because, if you ignore your feelings of hunger, you may end up eating too much later on.
- Eat your meals with others when you can and enjoy the social occasion.

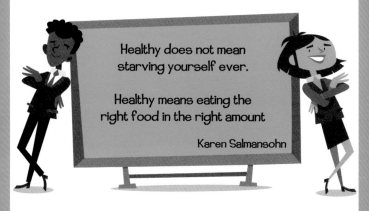

Healthy does not mean starving yourself ever.

Healthy means eating the right food in the right amount

Karen Salmansohn

Portion control

Food portion sizes today are far bigger than they have ever been, which means we are consuming a lot more calories than we sometimes realise. Many people no longer know what makes a normal portion. This is a problem with growing obesity statistics that is known as portion distortion.

You can better manage your portion size by following these 5 simple tips:

1. Eat with smaller plates and bowls.
2. Aim for two portions of vegetables on your plate to fill it with the healthiest option.
3. Eat slowly because it takes about 20 minutes for your stomach to tell your brain you are full.
4. Weigh your ingredients before you cook so you stick to the suggested serving sizes.
5. Drink a glass of water before you eat a meal.

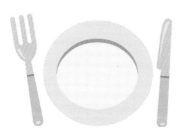

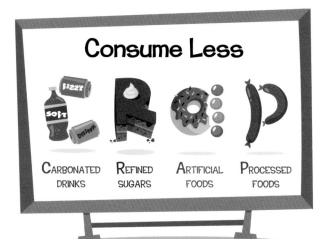

Refined sugar

Sugary foods can compromise your immune system. Research has shown that white blood cells are less efficient at fighting illness when exposed to refined sugar. A diet high in refined sugar will also raise your insulin levels quickly, which can lead to many other health problems. You will also lack energy as a result of these sugar spikes and the drop in blood sugar that follows.

The general advice is that you should have no more than 30 grams of free sugars a day, which is roughly equivalent to 7 sugar cubes. This is sugar that you add to your food. Choosing fresh fruits instead of sweet snacks such as biscuits, cakes and milk chocolate will help reduce consumption of sugars. You can also limit your intake of drinks high in sugars (fruit juices, cordials and syrups, flavoured milks and yogurt drinks) by switching to water.

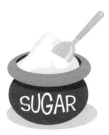

Salt

You may be unaware of the amount of salt you consume. The recommended level is less than 5 grams per day. That is about one teaspoon. Most salt comes from processed foods or from foods consumed frequently in large amounts like bread. Salt is also added to foods during cooking or at the point of consumption with table salt.

Salt intake can be reduced by:

- Limiting the amount of salt and high-sodium condiments you use when cooking and preparing foods.
- Not having salt or high-sodium sauces on the table.
- Limiting the consumption of salty snacks.
- Choosing products with lower sodium content.
- By consuming more potassium.

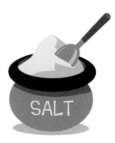

Good mood food

Keeping yourself healthy with a balanced diet can be good for your mental health and boost your mood too. If you are getting the right nutrients, your body will be better able to ward off anxiety during stressful times.

Here are a few useful foods that will boost your mood:

- Foods high in antioxidants such as blueberries and acai berries. These help to raise mood levels and lower the hormones responsible for stress.
- Foods that are high in vitamins D, B, and E, such as eggs, almonds and salmon.
- Foods high in omega-3 fatty acids, such as walnuts or flax seeds and oily fish.
- Foods high in minerals like magnesium, such as whole grains, green leafy vegetables, figs, avocados, bananas and raspberries, nuts and seeds, peas, broccoli, cabbage, green beans, artichokes, asparagus, seafood, salmon, mackerel and tuna.

NB – A lack of magnesium can result in a variety of symptoms, including anxiety.

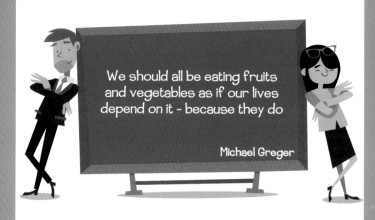

We should all be eating fruits and vegetables as if our lives depend on it - because they do

Michael Greger

Vegetables and fruit

People with diets rich in vegetables and fruit have a significantly lower risk of obesity, heart disease, stroke, diabetes and certain types of cancer. They are important sources of vitamins, minerals, dietary fibre, plant protein and antioxidants. It is important to eat a variety and especially leafy green vegetables because they are packed with vitamins, minerals and fibre and lower in calories.

It is recommended that you eat at least 5 portions of fruit and vegetables (excluding potatoes, sweet potatoes, cassava and other starchy roots) every day. A portion of fresh, canned or frozen fruit and vegetables is 80 grams. A portion of dried fruit is 30 grams. A 150ml glass of fruit juice, vegetable juice or smoothie also counts as one of your five-a-day, however limit the amount you have to no more than one glass a day.

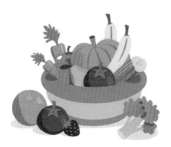

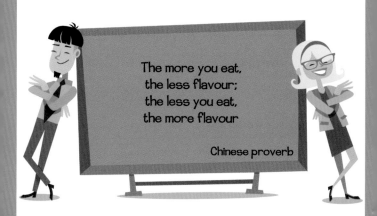

The more you eat,
the less flavour;
the less you eat,
the more flavour

Chinese proverb

Dark chocolate

There are nutrients in dark chocolate that can positively affect your health. One of the benefits of dark chocolate is that it is high in antioxidants, which are substances that can protect your cells, are anti-inflammatory and benefit the immune system.

Some studies show that diets high in antioxidants have many health benefits and, as part of a balanced and varied diet, dark chocolate can make a valuable contribution. The suggested cocoa content is between 70–80%. It is recommended to consume no more than 30 grams a day, and in excess of this you will end up putting on weight.

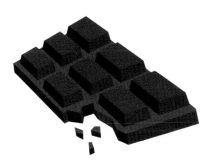

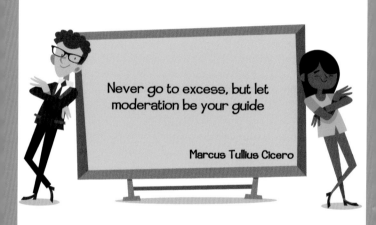

Never go to excess, but let moderation be your guide

Marcus Tullius Cicero

Drink alcohol in moderation

Excessive alcohol consumption can cause harm to your body's immune system in two ways. First of all, it can produce an overall nutritional deficiency, depriving your body of valuable immune-boosting nutrients. Secondly, alcohol, like sugar, consumed in excess can reduce the ability of white cells to kill germs and deplete your body of vitamin B, which can make you depressed.

Alcohol, despite the association with celebrations, is best enjoyed in moderation with the maximum recommended guidelines being 14 units a week for both men and women.

It is also recommended to have as many alcohol-free days a week as possible.

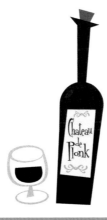

Keep hydrated

Water may not be the drink of choice, however keeping hydrated is one of the best things that you can do to keep healthy and it is vital for all bodily functions. An important part of flushing out bacteria is the actual flushing! Be planet friendly and use a reusable bottle and keep it with you at all times. Keep reminders around to ensure that you are drinking water throughout the day.

By keeping hydrated you will feel more alert and energised. There are lots of delicious herbal teas available and these will also add to your recommended quota of around two litres a day. There are over a billion people on this planet who don't have access to clean drinking water. We are extremely fortunate that we do!

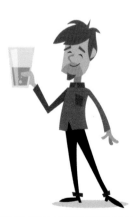

Caffeine

Caffeine is a stimulant found in tea, coffee, soft drinks, chocolate, kola nuts and some over-the-counter medicines. A cup of instant coffee can contain about 60 mg of caffeine; however, some commercially brewed coffee brands contain more than 150 mg of caffeine per serving.

Caffeine is recognised as an addictive substance by the World Health Organization (WHO). When consumed in moderate doses, caffeine can help people feel more alert and less sleepy. Currently, the general advice is not to consume more than 300 mg of caffeine a day. Too much coffee can make you feel anxious and disrupt sleep.

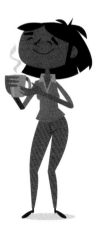

Weight management

A calorie is a unit that is used to measure energy and our bodies store and burn calories as fuel. Different types of food provide different levels of energy. When you eat and drink more calories than you use up, your body will store the excess as body fat.

As a guide, the average man needs 2500 calories a day and the average woman around 2000 calories. These values, however, will vary depending on age, size and levels of physical activity. To lose one pound of body fat you would need to burn 3500 calories. If you need to lose weight, the best approach is the following:

- Improve your knowledge of the calorific content of food.
- Reduce your intake by 500 calories a day.
- Reduce the amount of empty calories, which is food that has no nutritional content.
- Keep a log of what you are consuming.
- Increase your physical activity.
- Drink a glass of water when you get a hunger pang.

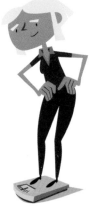

10 ways to strengthen your immune system

Following good-health guidelines is the best way that you can keep your immune system strong and healthy.

- Wash your hands frequently
- Eat a healthy balanced diet
- Exercise and relax regularly
- Maintain a healthy weight
- Reduce refined sugar
- Don't smoke
- Moderate alcohol consumption
- Make sure you get adequate sleep
- Manage and reduce stress levels
- Think positively and be kind

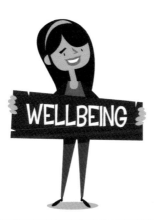

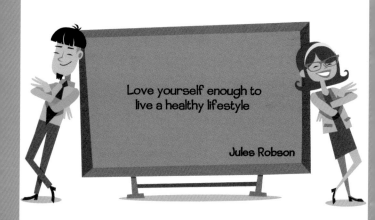

Love yourself enough to
live a healthy lifestyle

Jules Robson

Useful websites

If you are looking for more in-depth advice and don't know where to go, these websites have been helpful in researching this book. They have been curated for the excellent work they do in providing information about healthy eating.

- www.who.int/behealthy/healthy-diet
- www.who.int/news-room/fact-sheets/detail/healthy-diet
- www.thriveglobal.com/tags/healthy-eating/
- www.nhs.uk/live-well/eat-well/eight-tips-for-healthy-eating/
- www.heartuk.org.uk/tasty-recipes
- www.weightwatchers.com/
- www.nhs.uk/live-well/eat-well/
- www.nutrition.org.uk/healthyliving
- www.friendsoftheearth.uk/food
- www.bbcgoodfood.com

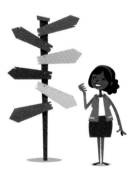

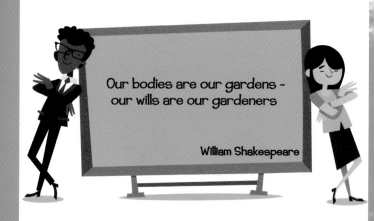

Our bodies are our gardens -
our wills are our gardeners

William Shakespeare